Disclaimer

This book is for informational purposes only and is not intended as medical advice, diagnosis or treatment. Always seek advice from a qualified physician about medical concerns and do not disregard medical advice because of something you may read within this book. This book does not replace the needs for diagnostic evaluation, ongoing physician care and professional assessment of treatments. Every effort has been made to make this book as complete and helpful as possible. It is important, however, for this book to be used as a resource and idea-generating guide and not as an ultimate source for plan of care.

ISBN 978-0-9910064-0-3

Copyright © 2013 by R.O.S. Therapy Systems, L.L.C.
All rights reserved including the right of reproduction in whole or in part.

Published by
R.O.S. Therapy Systems, L.L.C.
Greensboro, NC
888-352-9788
www.ROSTherapySystems.com

Activities 101 for the Family Caregiver

This book is a general guide to Activities for the Family Caregiver. It is based on the principles and approaches used in the training and certification of Professional Activity Directors in Long-Term Care settings. It is part of the complete R.O.S. package of Activities 101 books that will help you engage your senior loved one in meaningful activities.

With the assistance of Cindy Bradshaw and Dawn Appler-Worsley, who have been working in the field of Activities for Seniors for a combined 50 years, we have written this book for you in hope of providing helpful "How To's" for activities for your senior loved one.

We hope you find it useful and encourage you to have other family members and caregivers of your loved one read this in order to be consistent with approaches, verbal cues, physical assistance and modifications that produce positive results.

From our family of caregivers to yours, please remember that you are not alone and to never give up.

Scott Silknitter

Activities 101 Guidebook

Table of Contents

1. Activities, Benefits and the Family — 5

2. Communicating and Motivating for Success — 13

3. Planning and Executing Activities — 26

4. When Should I Do Activities? — 42

5. The "Lesson Plan" and Personal History — 50

6. Resources for Products and Education — 61

Family Members and Caregivers that have read this book:

_____

_____

_____

_____

_____

_____

_____

_____

_____

_____

Chapter 1

Activities, Benefits and the Family

"Activities" refers to any endeavor, other than routine Activities of Daily Living (ADLs), in which a senior participates. It is intended to enhance their sense of well-being and to promote or enhance physical, cognitive and emotional health.

The concept of using activities in a medical setting has origins in history as far back as the 1530s. Even Florence Nightingale gave advice to her nurses that discussed simple ideas on the delivery of activities. Nightingale went on to discuss the importance of using musical instruments and the use of small pets with patients for comfort and enjoyment.

In the institutional setting of today, "Activities" has grown into a profession where Certified Activity Professionals and their staff plan and execute Activity Programs for the residents and seniors in their care.

This guide was made for the millions of families and informal caregivers who care for seniors and their loved ones at home. It is based on the principles and approaches used by professionals.

A caregiver/family member's first priority is to deliver meaningful programs of interest to their loved one that focus on physical, social, spiritual, cognitive and recreational activities. Therapeutic programs can also promote self-reliance and provide opportunities for creativity, self-expression, self-satisfaction, fun and self-fulfillment. Some programs could specifically address managing stress, strengthening interpersonal skills, opportunities to learn new skills, or enhancing skills the senior already possesses.

The Benefits of Activities with a Standard Approach

Caregiver Benefit of Activities

Activities result in less stress for the caregiver as well as less stress for your senior. When your loved one is participating in activities, there will be less of a need to respond to behavioral issues. This will allow for more opportunities to engage positively with one another.

Social Benefit of Activities

Activities offer the opportunity for increased social interaction between family members, friends, caregivers and the one being cared for. Activities create positive experiences and memories for everyone.

Behavioral Benefit of Activities

Activities can reduce challenging behaviors when the activity conducted is interesting to your loved one. Offer activities at a skill level that allow your senior to enjoy the activity.

Self-Esteem Benefit of Activities

Activities offered at the right skill level provide your loved one with an opportunity for success. Success during activities improves how your loved one feels about themselves.

Sleep Benefit of Activities

As part of a daily routine, activities can improve sleeping at night. If a loved one is inactive all day, it is likely they will nap periodically. Napping can interrupt good sleep patterns at night.

Standard Approach Benefit of Activities

Being a primary caregiver is a 24/7 job. Without help, you are always on call and run the risk of becoming physically and mentally exhausted.

When you do bring in help, make sure all of your loved one's caregivers (full time, part time, family and friends) use the same approach for activities and interaction that you do. With a common approach, there are significantly less opportunities to disrupt routines and make unsettling changes that affect you and your loved one long after the help has left.

A common approach is key. Demand it!

Activities and the Family

It is critical to have as many family members involved in the senior's life as possible. Involvement not only shows the senior they are cared for and loved, but also gives the primary family caregiver the occasional break.

<u>Changes in Aging Families</u>

Almost every nation in the world is becoming progressively older. In just 100 years, the United States has gone from being a nation that consisted of primarily children to a nation primarily of adults. A couple of factors that have led to this transition include reduced fertility (women are having less babies) and reduced mortality (people are living longer).

Baby Boomers and Aging in Society

The baby boom represents over 76 million babies who were born between 1946 and 1964. Baby boomers as a generation do not like to talk about their demise and in turn are in denial and avoid discussing their long-term plans.

Demographic and Social Changes in Families

Social and historical changes in the structure of families have strongly influenced the functions of intergenerational relationships.

Chapter 1 Notes

Chapter 2

Communicating and Motivating for Success

Communicating is vital to the success of an activity with your senior. The key to effective communication is the ability to listen attentively. This requires the caregiver to use communication techniques that provide an open, nonthreatening environment for your senior. Listening behavior can either enhance and encourage communication or shut down communication altogether. People need to assess their listening style as well as be able to assess the listening styles of other caregivers and family members working with your senior.

Verbal Communication

Communication is an interactive process where information is exchanged. The ability to respond appropriately, to give feedback on something that was communicated, is just as important as good listening skills.

Verbal Approaches

- Use exact, short, positive phrases. Repeat twice if necessary.
- Speak slowly. Give time for the person to answer. Give one instruction at a time.
- Use a warm, gentle tone of voice.
- Talk to them like an adult.
- Only use words that the senior is familiar with.

Nonverbal Communication

Although it may seem that most communication happens verbally, research has shown that most communication occurs nonverbally. Nonverbal communication occurs through an individual's body language. There are five key elements to consider:

Facial Expressions

Be aware what your facial expressions are conveying to a senior. Remember, your mood will be mirrored.

Eye Contact

Ensure you have eye contact and that the senior is focused on you and what you are saying.

Gestures and Touch

Use nonverbal signs such as pointing and waving, along with using universal gestures in combination with your words.

Tone of Voice

The inflection in your voice helps your senior relate to the words you are saying.

Body Language

Be aware of the position of your hands and arms when talking to your loved one.

Nonverbal Approaches

- Always approach the senior from the front before speaking.
- Smile and extend your hand as to shake their hand. Use touch where welcomed.
- Get eye level with the person you are talking to.
- Use nonverbal gestures along with words. Give nonverbal praises such as smiles and head nods.

Approaches to Successful Communication

Be Calm

Always approach the senior in a relaxed and calm demeanor. Your mood will be mirrored by the senior. Smiles are contagious.

Be Flexible

There is no right or wrong way of completing a task. Offer praise and encouragement for the effort the senior puts into a task. If you see the senior becoming overwhelmed or frustrated, stop the task and re-approach at another time.

Be Nonresistive

Don't force tasks on the senior. Adults do not want to be told, "No!" or told what to do. The power of suggestion goes a long way.

Be Guiding but Not Controlling

Always use a soft, gentle approach. Remember your tone of voice. Your facial expressions must match the words you are saying.

Barriers to Good Communication

There are generally two barriers that negatively affect communication with your senior. Here are some tips on how to eliminate those:

Barriers Created by Caregivers

- Slow down when speaking. Use a calm tone of voice and be aware of your hand movements.
- Never be demanding or commanding.
- Never argue with a person with impaired cognition. You will never win the argument.
- Enter their world. Live their truth.
- Do not ask memory questions.
- Do not offer long explanations when answering questions.

Environmental Barriers to Communication

- Air conditioners and home appliances
- TV on in the same room where you are trying to talk
- Outside traffic
- Hearing aid battery that is whistling

Validation of "Living their Truth" as a Tool to Good Communication

Our role when working with a senior is best expressed by author Jolene Brackey, who preaches that caregivers should take every opportunity to create moments of joy.

Many people struggle with the use of validation because it could appear as if you are lying to a senior or doing a senior harm by not keeping them oriented to the truth. You are not lying to the senior. You are meeting the senior where they are for the moment and accepting that this is part of the illness.

Communication and Behavior

Behaviors are a means to communicate when words are no longer effective. Caregivers must uncover the meaning behind the behaviors and put a plan into effect to manage those needs. Your job is to uncover the meaning or causes behind the behaviors.

Repetitive Behaviors

Repetitive behavior can manifest itself as repetitive movements, sounds and words. Typical repetitive behaviors could be repetitive questions, words or phrases, clapping or rubbing of the hands, pacing, often accompanied by dusting or wiping motion or rummaging through drawers and closets.

Aggressive Behaviors

Aggressive behavior can be defined as hitting, angry outburst, obscenities, yelling, racial insults, sexual comments and/or biting. It can be fearful for a caregiver to communicate or provide care to a senior who is aggressive.

Possible Causes for Aggression

- Too much noise/over stimulation
- Cluttered environment or uncomfortable temperatures
- Basic needs not being met: Hungry, thirsty, need bathroom, need comfort
- Pain
- Fear/anxiety/confusion
- Communication barriers
- Scared that they do not recognize their surroundings
- Caregiver's mood
- Senior perceives that they are being rushed

Interventions to Utilize with a Senior with Aggressive Behaviors

- Communicate for success.
- Reminisce with the senior about specific details of their past.
- Validate and support their feelings.
- Find items that they find comfort in, i.e. a photograph of the family.
- Provide consistent caregivers and a consistent schedule. Stick to the senior's routine.
- Provide recreational activities that match their abilities and interests, as tolerated.
- Break down instructions into one step increments.
- Identify the triggers of the aggression. Be a detective. There is never a behavior that just occurs.
- Keep ongoing communication between family members and caregivers over any noted changes in patterns or behaviors.
- Help the senior to slow down and relax.

- Use music to calm the seniors (providing they like music and ensure it matches their interest).
- Use spiritual support if this is important to the senior.
- Remain calm and speak in a soft tone.
- Utilize the R.O.S. Therapy Systems products, activity board inserts, R.O.S. BIG Book, and R.O.S. Theme Books.

Chapter 2 Notes

Chapter 3

Planning and Executing Activities

Activities are generally broken down into three different areas:

Maintenance Activities

These are traditional activities that help a senior to maintain physical, cognitive, social, spiritual and emotional health.

Supportive Activities

For those types of seniors that have a lower tolerance for traditional activities, these types of activities provide a comfortable environment while providing stimulation or solace.

Empowering Activities

These are activities that help a senior attain self-respect by receiving opportunities for self-expression and responsibility.

To start, determine which types of activities should be performed with your senior. Then you must look at their functional level through an assessment.

Functional Levels

When planning meaningful activities based on an individual's needs and interests, it is first good to assess their functional ability. There are several definitions of functional levels. For the purposes of this topic, we will address the following four functioning levels:

Level 1

The senior has good social skills. They are able to communicate. They are alert and oriented to person, place and time, and they have a long attention span.

Level 2

The senior has less social skills and their verbal skills may be impaired as well. The senior may have some behavior symptoms. They may need something to do, and may have an increased energy level, yet a shorter attention span.

Level 3

The senior has less social skills. Their verbal skills are even more impaired than they were at Level 2 and they are distracted easily. The senior may have some visual/spatial perception and balance concerns and they need maximum assistance with their care.

Level 4

The senior has a low energy level, nonverbal skills, and they rarely initiate contact with others, however, they may respond if given time and cues.

Information Gathering and Assessment

Knowing your senior's individual needs, interests, functional abilities and capacities will assist you in knowing how to plan and engage in meaningful, quality leisure activities. As the primary caregiver, you probably already know the answers, but this is a good and necessary exercise for you, other family members and other caregivers to execute. The following types of informal information can be gathered from your senior:

Basic Information

Name, preferred name to be called, age and date of birth

Background Information

Place of birth, cultural/ethnic background, marital status, children (how many, and their names), religion/church, military service/employment, education level and primary language spoken

Medical and Dietary/Nutritional Information

Any formal diagnosis, allergies and food regiment/diets

Habits

Drinking/alcohol, smoking, exercise and other things that are a daily habit

Physical Status

Abilities/limitations, visual aids, hearing deficits, speech, communication, hand dominance and mobility/gait

Mental Status

Alertness, cognitive abilities/limitations, orientation to family, time, place, person, routine, etc.

Social Status/Preferences

One-on-one interaction, being visited, communication with others through written words, phone calls or other means

Emotional Status

Content, outgoing, introvert, withdrawn, dependent/independent

Leisure Status

Past, present and future interests

Informal Assessments

Informal assessments are done through interviews, observation, and information gathered through other means.

Interviews

These are conducted with either the senior or with family members, friends or significant others.

Observation

This is what is seen or observed during the initial meeting phase. What is seen or heard concerning the senior? How do they interact with others? How is their behavior and response to questions or statements made by others? Body language and expressions would also be observed during the initial contact and thereafter.

Information Gathered Through Other Means

Request family members or friends help complete a history of the senior to assist with getting to know them better.

Formal Assessments

Formal assessments measure specific functional abilities such as physical, cognitive, emotional and social skills. They are also utilized to assess self-esteem, coping skills, stress levels, interests and other things that could be barriers to successful participation in leisure activities.

NOTE: The person that conducts these formal assessments needs to be trained in order for them to be administered, scored and read correctly.

Activity Treatment Potential

After the senior has been interviewed for their interests, and their functional ability has been assessed, development of an activity plan can commence.

Through the assessment process, you have gathered all types of information about the types of activities you will initiate with your senior. Keeping in mind their limitations, if applicable, the focus throughout the assessment should be to develop activities that offer the senior their maximum potential to work at their highest practical level of functioning whether physically, socially, cognitively or creatively.

<u>Physically</u>

Rather than maintaining the individual's current level of activity, encourage them to work at their highest level.

Socially

If the senior wants to communicate with their loved ones or friends, rather than dictating a letter to you as the caregiver to be written, perhaps the senior could write their own words, or utilize a computer to send an email, or even encourage them to Skype™ or utilize some other technology to challenge their social abilities.

Cognitively

The more a senior thinks for themselves, the more they will stay alert and oriented.

Creatively

Encourage them to pick their own colors, their own techniques and give them the tools to augment the best possible outcome.

We are human and all have a need to be productive and purposeful. You, the family caregiver, must find what your senior's motivator is and then give the senior a reason that makes sense to them as to why they should be active.

Best Practices for Engaging a Senior with Dementia

- Have a Personal History Interview completed.
- Activities should be person appropriate.
- Redefine your idea of, "What is an activity program?"
- Active activities can include: Baking, basketball, taking a walk, etc.
- Passive activities can include: Arranging flowers, Bible stories, bubbles, etc.
- Memory boxes. Examples for theme boxes include:
  - *Art box* – Paint brushes, canvas boards, finished paintings, drawings and colored pencils. You can ask the senior to tell you what these items are and what they are used for.

- *Baby Box* – Baby clothes, baby dolls, diapers, baby booties, stuffed animals, lotion, music box, baby blanket.
- *Jewelry Box* – Can be costume jewelry if you are concerned about having your family heirlooms and valuables accessible.
- Reminiscing Box – Specific items that are mementoes of the person, photographs, and collectables that they have treasured throughout their life.

Programming for Individuals with Mild to Moderate Dementia

Many seniors have cognitive deficits that are significant enough to impact their day as well as their awareness of their surroundings. By providing activities that reinforce their past, we increase and improve their social skills which can improve their general interactions with others.

Validating Activities

These activities validate the memories and feelings of individuals who are much disoriented. They focus on the senior's perception of what happened in the past. Naomi Feil, founder of validation methods, does not focus on orientation, but rather a person's perception of what happened in their past.

Reminiscing Activities

Reminiscing activities are designed to help the client identify the important contributions he or she has made throughout their lifetime. It is an important part of human development to see oneself as a contributing member of society.

Resocializing Activities

Once your senior can successfully participate in reminiscing and validating activities, it is time to encourage them to build on those social skills and begin to expand their connections to the community in which they live. This can be as simple as with a neighbor, in church, or within their community.

Topics for Engaging a Senior with Dementia

- Colors
- Favorite Music
- War Stories
- Holidays
- Home Cooking
- Sports
- School Days
- Old Cars
- Any Information obtained from their Personal History Assessment Interview

NOTE: As dementia progresses, parts of the brain die along with memories and abilities controlled by the parts of the brain. An 80-year-old may have memories and abilities of a 7-year-old.

Engaging Activities
with Someone who has Difficult Behaviors

- Reduce Noise and Visual Distractions
  - ° Make sure you have your senior's attention when speaking.

- Increase Environmental Cues
  - ° Ensure your senior has proper lighting to see what they are doing.

- Maintain each Senior's Normal Schedule as Much as Possible
  - ° Keeping a consistent schedule with their daily routine will provide your senior a sense of security. A weekday schedule should look the same as a weekend schedule.

Chapter 3 Notes

Chapter 4

When Should I Do Activities?

Activities occur all day every day. The question should not be, "When should I do activities?" It is not important to focus on when to do activities. The focus should be on making each and every interaction memorable and always focusing on the senior as an individual.

Person Appropriate

Person appropriate refers to the idea that each person has a personal identity and history. Let's use gardening as an example of an activity. Person appropriate could mean different things to different people. Four people might all say they like gardening during their assessment, yet might not enjoy the same activity. The following page gives us examples of four people that like gardening, but each have a different thought of what gardening means to them.

- Person 1 – Would only enjoy going outside, cutting the grass, trimming the hedges and weed whacking. Anything less would not meet their preference.

- Person 2 – Enjoys getting in the flowerbeds, planting flowers and vegetables, and tending to their garden on their hands and knees each day for an hour.

- Person 3 – Enjoys indoor plants. Enjoys propagating plants and watering and caring for plants daily.

- Person 4 – Enjoys arranging flowers in vases for tables.

You can tell by the above example, one specific activity does not meet the interest of every individual and, therefore, when planning activities, you need to ensure the activity is person appropriate.

Customary Routines and Preferences

For the purpose of developing a daily plan of care, we will be discussing two areas: Daily Customary Routine and Activity Preferences. The goal is to gain from the senior's perspective how important certain aspects of care/activity are of interest to them as an individual.

Daily Customary Routine

Your senior has distinct lifestyle preferences and they should be preserved to the extent possible. All reasonable accommodation should be made to maintain their lifestyle preferences.

Not accommodating your senior's lifestyle preferences can contribute to depressed mood and increased behavior symptoms. When a person feels like their control has been removed and that their preferences are not respected as an individual, it can be demoralizing.

Activity Preferences

Activities are a way for individuals to establish meaning in their lives. The need for enjoyable activities does not change based on their age or health needs. The only thing that changes is the level of assistance they may need to engage in those pursuits.

A lack of opportunity to engage in meaningful and enjoyable activities can result in boredom, depression and behavioral disturbances.

Individuals vary in the activities they prefer, reflecting unique personalities, past interest, perceived environmental constraints, religious and cultural background, and changing physical and mental abilities. We as family caregivers have a great opportunity to empower a senior to see that they possess many great talents and abilities. By modifying or adapting an activity to allow them to engage at an independent level, you are restoring their self-esteem and self-worth.

Activity Programming Related to Medical Care Areas

Activity engagement encompasses much more than to keep one occupied throughout the day. Activities are an important therapeutic modality in the healthcare that is provided. An ongoing meaningful activity program can help address, redirect or eliminate many medical conditions.

Delirium

An acute confused state, delirium is a syndrome that presents as severe confusion and disorientation, developing with relatively rapid onset and fluctuation in intensity. It is a syndrome which occurs more frequently in people in their later years.

Cognitive Loss/Dementia

Cognitive loss/dementia activities provide positive experiences that are modified to the individual's abilities.

They help the senior participate at their highest practical level.

Communication Barriers

Use nonverbal communication along with the spoken word.

Psychosocial Well-Being

During every interaction we have with a senior we must ask ourselves, "How does this affect their psychosocial well-being?" This includes words you choose in response to the type of interactions and activities that are provided.

Depressed Mood

If you are consistent with your approaches, utilize the life review to individualize an activity program, and then modify and adapt each activity to promote independence, you are less likely to have a senior with a depressed mood. Have your senior tell their story.

Behaviors

Keep in mind that behaviors are nothing more than a means to communicate. When faced with a difficult behavior, develop a behavior management plan that can be utilized consistently with family and caregivers. Introduce activities that will teach coping skills, relaxation and anger management techniques. Keep activities short in duration and repetition.

Chapter 4 Notes

Chapter 5

The "Lesson Plan" and Personal History

The "Lesson Plan" template is a guideline for an activity. Each senior's abilities and responses are different. This will dictate how you modify an activity to meet their individual needs and abilities. The lesson plan is an ever-changing document. It is meant to be written on to note any changes you made in the original lesson plan so the family member or the caregiver working with your senior next can follow your modifications in hopes to recreate a positive experience.

Items in the Lesson Plan

<u>Date</u>

Document the date the program is used with your senior.

Program Name

You can rename the program if your senior prefers.

Objective of Activity

Our goal is to provide meaningful activities. People have a need to be productive and they want to engage in something with a purpose. List the objectives of the program.

Materials

The list of suggested materials to use with this program.

Prerequisite Skills

The skills your senior needs to participate in this program.

Activity Outline

Step-by-step instructions to complete this program.

Evaluation

When you or a family member are conducting an activity with the senior, documenting results and responses are critical to improve activity programs for your senior. Items to document:

- Verbal cues, physical assistance or modifications you make to activity.
- Your senior's response to this program.
- Did your senior enjoy this activity or not?
- Was the activity successful at distracting or eliminating a negative behavior?

A blank template is included on the next page to give you an example of what a template looks like.

NOTE: Make sure caregivers and family members are consistent with the type of verbal cues, physical assistance or modifications that produce positive results.

Lesson Plan Blank Template

Date:	Program Name:
Objective of Activity	
➢ ➢ ➢	
Materials	
➢ ➢ ➢	
Prerequisite Skills	
➢ ➢ ➢	
Activity Outline	
Evaluation	

Chapter 5 Notes

This is _____ *'s Personal History*

Name:

Maiden Name:

Date of Birth:

Preferred Name:

Name and relationship of people completing this history:

What age do you think the person thinks they are?

Do they ask for their spouse but do not recognize them?

Do they look for their children but do not recognize them?

Do they look for their mom?

Do they perceive themselves as younger? Please describe:

Describe the "home" they remember.

Describe the person's personality prior to the onset of the disease.

What makes the person feel valued? Talents, occupation, accomplishments, family, etc.

What are some favorite items they must always have in sight or close by?

What is their exact morning routine?

What is their exact evening routine?

Type of clothing they prefer and do they like to choose their clothing or have it laid out for them?

What is their favorite beverage?

What is their favorite food?

What will get them motivated? Church, friends coming over, going out, etc.

List significant interests in their life: Hobbies, recreational, job related, military, etc.

    - Age 8 to 20:

- Age 20 to 40:

Religious background? Affiliation, prayer time, symbols, traditions, church name, etc.

What type of music do they like? Give examples of any musical talents.

What is their favorite TV program? Movie?

Can he / she tell the difference between someone on TV and a real person?

Marital status - If married more than once, give specifics. Include: Names, dates and relevant information.

List distinct characteristics about your senior's spouse: Occupation, personality or daily routine.

Does he /she have children? If yes, give names, birth dates and any relevant information.

Who do they ask for the most? What is their relationship? Describe how that person spends their day.

What causes stress to them?

What calms them down when stressed or agitated?

Other information that would help bring joy to your senior.

Resources for Products and Education

R.O.S. Therapy Systems – The mission of R.O.S. Therapy Systems is to improve quality of life through entertainment and activities.
www.ROSTherapySystems.com
Toll-Free: 888-352-9788
Email: info@ROSTherapySystems.com

Alzheimer's Association – The Alzheimer's Association works on a global, national and local level to enhance care and support for all those affected by Alzheimer's and related dementias.
www.alz.org
Toll-Free: 800-272-3900
Email: info@alz.org

National Parkinson Foundation – The mission of the National Parkinson Foundation is simple — to improve the lives of people with Parkinson's disease through research, education and outreach.
www.parkinson.org
Toll-Free: 800-4PD-INFO (473-4636)
Email: contact@parkinson.org

Lewy Body Dementia Association – (LBDA) is a 501(c)(3) nonprofit organization dedicated to raising awareness of the Lewy body dementias (LBD), supporting people with LBD, their families and caregivers and promoting scientific advances. The Association's purposes are charitable, educational and scientific.

www.lbda.org
Toll-Free: 800-539-9767

National Certification Council of Activity Professionals – (NCCAP) – The National Certification Council for Activity Professionals (NCCAP) is one of the Certifying Bodies recognized by Federal law and incorporated in many state regulations. NCCAP is the ONLY national organization that exclusively certifies activity professionals who work with the elderly.

www.nccap.org
Phone: 757-552-0653
Email: info@nccap.org

About The Authors

Dawn Appler-Worsley, ADC/EDU/U/MC, CDP

Dawn Appler-Worsley is a Certified Activity Director with a specialization in Education and Memory Care, a Certified Eden Alternative Associate and a Certified Dementia Practitioner. With over 20 years of experience, Ms. Appler-Worsley is an authorized certification instructor with the National Certification Council of Dementia Practitioners and a Modular Education Program for Activity Professionals course instructor.

Cindy Bradshaw, MS, ACC

With a 30-year career in Geriatrics, a BS Human Services and Gerontology, and as the Executive Director of National Certification Council for Activity Professionals, Ms. Bradshaw is a leader in the field of activities. She co-developed and teaches the Modular Education Program for Activity Professionals (MEPAP 2nd Edition) by which Activity Professionals are certified to.

Scott Silknitter

Scott Silknitter is the founder of R.O.S. Therapy Systems. He designed and created the R.O.S. Play Therapy™ System, the *How Much Do You Know About* Series of themed activity books and the R.O.S. BIG Book Subscription. Starting with a simple backyard project to help Mom and Dad, Mr. Silknitter has dedicated his life to improving the quality of life for all seniors through entertainment and activities.

References
1. The Handbook of Theories on Aging (Bengtson et al., 2009)
2. Activity Keeps Me Going, Volume A, (Peckham et al., 2011)
3. Essentials for the Activity Professional in Long-Term Care (Lanza, 1997)
4. Abnormal Psychology, Butcher
5. The Wind and the SunÆsop. (Sixth century B.C.) Fables. The Harvard Classics. 1909–14.
6. info@dhspecialservices.com*book 2)
7. National Certification Council for Dementia Practitioners www.NCCDP.org
8. Managing Difficult Dementia Behaviors: An A-B-C Approach By Carrie Steckl
9. Iowa Geriatric Education Center website, Marianne Smith, PhD, ARNP, BC Assistant Professor University of Iowa College of Nursing
10. *Excerpts taken from "Behavior...Whose Problem is it?" Hommel, 2012
11. Merriam-Webster's dictionary
12. The Latent Kin Matrix (Riley, 1983)
13. CarePlanning Cookbook (Nolta et al.2007)
14. Long-Term Care (Blasko et al. 2011)
15. Success Oriented Programs for the Dementia Client (Worsley et al 2005)
16. Heerema, Esther. "Eight Reasons Why Meaningful Activities Are Important for People with Dementia." www.about.com